The really, really, really useful

Guide.

Number 5

MAKE-UP
REVEALED

MIKE PEARCE

DEDICATION

This book is dedicated to all those who use or do not use make-up, especially those just thinking of doing so. It is also dedicated to those who need make-up in their jobs or roles in life to bring enjoyment and something special to their character and lifestyle.

CONTENTS

Acknowledgments

ACKNOWLEDGMENTS

The author would like to thank Rebecca Pearce for checking the manuscript. Also, to all those who cheered and clapped me when walking through the streets in the Dickens' Parade in Rochester and Broadstairs for the last 20 years heavily chained and with make-up appropriate for someone who has just returned from the dead to haunt Ebenezer Scrooge.

THE OLD WOMAN (Joseph Campbell)

As a white candle

In a holy place

So is the beauty

Of an aged face

This book looks at a brief history of make-up and its use. It also gives the terminology used in make-up as well as the phrases that can encourage you to spend tens if not hundreds of pounds. Many people do not even look at what is on the packaging and most people have no idea what the chemicals are that will soon be adorning their face. Some recognisable ingredients such as fruits and plant oils taken from aromatherapy have been used to soften this ignorance. Many ingredients used in the past caused more damage than beneficial effect and still today some chemicals can still be rated as questionable. Some professions require a person to wear make-up which is unavoidable but minimum make-up for others is closest to beauty and remember most people choose inner beauty not physical attractiveness when choosing their partner.

1 INTRODUCTION

When a person reaches twenty five years old collagen and elastin production decreases so the skin in the face can lose its firmness and tone, also its smoothness due to less oil production. People have looked for natural substances and now manufactured chemicals to hide this effect which gave rise to the terms 'make-up' and 'cosmetics'. Make-up is a term initially used from 1870. This word in the Oxford dictionary gives examples such as lipstick or powder which one applies to the face to enhance or alter the appearance. Cosmetics initially referred to things applied medically. Kosmos means to arrange, order or adorn. The word cosmetic is wider referring to a preparation applied to the body and especially the face to improve one's appearance.

Plantus a Roman writer said "A woman without paint is like food without salt".

Symmetrical faces have always been more attractive. For example the Egyptian Queen and chief consort of the pharaoh Akhenaten, Nefertiti, is considered by some to be the most beautiful woman in the world.

Make-up used to pinken cheeks and redden lips mimics the increased blood flow in face and lips during ovulation. The hormone shift at this time makes women seem more available and more attractive. Adding black make-up mimics mid -cycle ovulation. Darkening eyes or lips makes one seem more attractive, and shiny, wet, bright lips indicate arousal.

Women also put on make-up try to regain the pretty childlike look. Healthy pink cheeks indicate youth. Trying to make your eyes bigger mimics the typical face of a young child. Babies, like young animals and those appealing cartoon animal characters, always have large eyes and big eyelashes. Today people use eyeliners, eye shadow and mascara to get these large eyes, and lipstick and lip liners to get the large lips of the baby face. Full eyebrows also can indicate youth.

Make-up especially in the past was used to hide imperfections and to cover up disease or disfigurement. Layers of powder and paint were put on the face and this in itself could cause more damage, being toxic or causing allergic reactions. Some preparations still used today can cause similar problems.

2 HISTORY

- Body paint can go back to 400,000 years plus it is believed

- The Egyptians were the first people to use make-up seriously. Eyeliner was used in 10,000BC in ancient Egypt, Mesopotamia

- Ancient Egyptians used Kohl which was lead sulphide and soot to paint faces. This was used around the rim of the eyes of all the family including the children. It was believed, as was the other make-up used to protect against the ultraviolet rays from the sun. The Egyptians liked make-up which was red, blue, black and magenta. Some people had cones of perfumed grease above their faces in their hair which melted in the hot climate and ran down and cooled them in the process

- Egyptian eye make-up was also thought to prevent infection and the Gods Horus and Ra would protect them against disease. Eyeliner was used to protect eyes from the Sun God and also to ward off the Evil Eye. Lipstick could be made from carmine beetles and applied using wet sticks of wood

- Cleopatra used black galena for her eyebrows. Her upper eyelids were deep blue and her lower eyelids were bright green. Men and women in Egypt painted kohl around their eyes, often made from lead sulphide then they changed to charcoal or soot.

- The Aztecs used cochineal as dye for lip and eyes

- Some Ancient Greeks used ox hair for eyebrows

- Ancient Rome and Greece thought you looked sickly or unattractive wearing make-up but one kind of make-up was used by both courtesans male and female

- Romans of higher status wore more make-up and used red ochre eye shadow made from saffron. Eye paint was red, and black was popular. Lead tetroxide and mercuric sulphur were commonly used

- Some Roman women used crocodile dung for face packs, and they used a cream made of beeswax, olive oil and rosewater with clay. Romans also painted their lips to show rank while for anti-ageing used proteinaceous snail slime, ashes, and swan fat could fill up the wrinkles

- In the Middle Ages the Catholic Church believed that make-up was sinful.

- Medieval 15th century women used bat's blood to redden their face

- Coal tar was used on the eyes in Elizabethan times and this caused blindness

- Sixteenth-century beautification involved red lips and red cheeks, with Kohl to make eyes look larger and further set apart. Also, eye brows were plucked and eyebrows raised. In the 16th century Mona Lisa had plucked eyebrows as that was the fashion

- The seventeenth century lower and middle classes did not have the money or time to wear make-up but they still did so in court. As make-up could cause scar and lesions they would wear face patches.

- In the late 1700's men came back from the Grand Tour and brought with them not only with them fashion but also increased the use of make-up. These were nicknamed Macaroni's as referred to in the classic nursery rhyme-Yankee Doodle went to town, Riding on a Pony, Stuck a feather in his cap, and called him Macaroni.

- In the 18th century even children wore make-up to match their social status. Even middle classes would whiten their faces with white lead and would use large circles of red rouge on their cheeks. They also darkened their eyebrows and covered their freckles as well as using jars of cold cream. The trend then changed to using zinc oxide for whitening as it was safer.

- Women commonly used a mixture of white lead and egg and vinegar on their faces and neck to pale their skin and to cover blemishes. White faces indicated higher status than the labourers whose faces were darkened by working in the fields.

- The eighteenth century paleness was even more important for both men and women in court and they shaved their eyebrows, replacing them with fur from grey mice stuck on above their eyes. Women could be Leeched the bleeding lightening their faces

- Around the French revolution rouge, black and silk beauty spots were more common. Different shaped or position of beauty spots could have a meaning. If they were placed at the corner of the eye you were a passionate person, on the forehead indicated majesty while on the nose suggested sauciness. In London parliament right wing wigs had their beauty spot on the right cheek while left wing Tories had theirs on the left.

- Clergymen preached after the French Revolution against painted ladies. They were despised by the church and Victorians in the 18th century could divorce their wife for having make-up on. Women used to pinch their face to get red cheeks before blush or rouge was invented. In the 18th century lead poisoning was common, eyes became inflamed and the skin went black.

- At 18th century court in France they wanted white skin so they applied thick layers of white powdered lead, talc and bone. Blue lines were drawn to represent veins.

- In the 1850s they used cold crème made from wax from whales, almond oil, and rose water. 18th Century Americans used warm young boy's urine to remove freckles.

- During the 1880s and in the Naughty Ninety's make-up flourished.

- Queen Victoria wanted modesty in the 19th century. Queen Victoria declared that make-up was improper and vulgar and should only be used by actors.

- Edwardian make-up was mainly related to stage activities. The pale look was still fashionable and lemon juice was put on the face. Rouge was used for cheeks and lips. Lavender powder would lighten faces in candle light.

- A lot of DIY dyes were added to make-up. Egg white was used to conceal wrinkles; ochre gave a reddish for cheeks and carmine for lips.

- To hide freckles they used rice powder, zinc oxide, pearl powder, and expensive zinc oxide.

- Crushed flowers were used for lips. Carmine from cochineal insects was used and also beetroot for cheeks. For eyes, lemon juice or orange was to clean them. Belladonna dilated eyes and was used for cataracts. Beeswax was put on the eyelashes mixed with soot, and applied with burnt hair pins.

- In 1909, women visiting Selfridges
  experimented with cosmetics as did the Max
  Factor group. By 1910 the market had
  developed and rouge could now be used for
  lips, cheeks and the forehead. Previously,
  mascara could be made using vaseline and
  soot. Then proper cake mascara was
  developed by Eugene Rimmel and by 1916
  false eyelashes were used in films. Lipsticks, a
  few years later were developed into sticks and
  then held in swivel containers.
  By the end of the Roaring Twenties over three
  thousand face powders were available and
  hundreds of rouges

- During World War 2 there was a limit on
  cosmetics except lipstick which was boosted
  by Winston Churchill so that more nurses
  looked like women. Red Lipstick would
  remind the troops that they were ladies as well
  as nurses.

- With new medical treatments available for
  face problems less make-up was needed for

cover up but still eyebrows and lips were exaggerated

- After the Second World War with the lack of cosmetics this produced many new commercial companies. Initially, many people just used soap and water and a pot of face cream but in Hollywood lots of famous names set the trend in make-up use and by the 1950s many women used lipstick and rouge. As in the forties screen stars wore bright lipsticks.

- A move through the 70's, 80's and 90's was to try and obtain the natural look and face powders became made up of very fine particles.

- By the 1960s-70s feminism arose and cosmetics were not worn by many women so as not to be seen as sex objects. Softer lipsticks, eyeliners and eyeshadows were preferred to darker ones. Red, blue and green make-up was especially popular and mascara was still being applied with a wet brush. False eyelashes and heavy eyeliner came into use.

- Lipliner was in favour and powders were used less. Models, advertising and magazines had a huge influence on purchase of make-up as well as major block buster movies such as Cleopatra. Electrical massage was carried out with face masks. Fake tan was being used but it was not realistic as it could be dark or produce orange streaks.

- In the 1980s skin care was emphasised, together with anti-ageing products and the dangers of too much time in the sun. Non-invasive facial treatments as used by celebrities were popular. Botox based on a botulism product, was being used and it would paralyse the face muscles. Also, collagen implants were coming in to help produce pouting lips and to remove lines and wrinkles

- From then on manufacturers looked at the need of non-western cultures especially in the world of skin care, and online channels have helped increase world markets.

- Today's wearers need time saving and long lasting formulations which incorporate as many kinds of skin care as possible, e.g. protection from the sun. Today anyone, any sex, can use make-up. Make-up often is waterproof in rain or during crying; it doesn't crack or wear off too soon but has an added advantage of it being a professional skin treatment. Cost also is important and online shopping has helped to reduce some prices and web sites provide different choices. Legislation has for some products helped select environmentally friendly products and safer ones.

3 TO USE OR NOT TO USE

- Acts as a mask to hide behind
- Adverts show good looking women which society likes
- A great range of colour like a paint box to play with and use your artistic talent
- Becomes a ritual-'Just put on a bit of lippy before a meeting'
- Can disguise disfigurement and shade skin from the sun
- Can make you look like a doll or create a baby face which is more attractive
- Can pose a threat to other women with a lot of make-up on
- Can send a message through colours or geometrical designs
- Can sculpture faces using bronze, skin highlighters and dark pigment
- Can think yourself unattractive without it

- Can use exotic colours -emerald green. leaf or apple green, violet, deep reds and canary yellow. Vintage look
- Contouring of face is more important in women
- Don't like blemishes, can use make-up to cover them up.
- Enhances your best facial features
- Enhances your emotions
- Empowers you
- Feel good factor
- Feel nude without it because other women wear it. Can also get smoky nude colour.
- Female skin is lighter than men's skin
- Friends use it so they have the highest influence
- Get paid more by wearing make-up
- Girls can be jealous of those wearing lot of make-up
- Gives confidence
- Good looking skin denotes health
- Have a bias towards childlike proportions

- Helps self esteem
- Helps to attract a partner/mate. Part of being a woman
- Helps to give you power
- Helps you win elections
- Ill health has made the texture of your skin look like clay or lifeless
- Just looking at the packaging can make you feel good
- Keep men happy daily
- Lighter skin suggests youthfulness but darker skin comes with age
- Lipstick is more attractive to men especially a red colour
- Makes you seem more competent and likeable
- Make-up helps people to see your expressions from a distance
- Make-up can make the difference between getting and not getting a job at interview but lesser make-up can indicate a professional
- Make-up is art, you can use colour sparkle and shine

- Males have more contrast between their eyes and they stand out more so don't need the same make up.
- Women have to have make-up to stand out.
- May feel bad if not wearing it
- More make-up the more money, i.e. assume richer people are wasting money on make-up
- Not taken seriously at work without it. It may be even be compulsory.
- Old grannies look younger with make-up
- Only way you can express yourself
- Part of being a woman
- People judge you when they look at you
- Putting on make-up on becomes a habit.
- Recognised as feminine
- Skin care is more noticeable if you use make-up
- Some ingredients are good for skin
- To attract attention
- To indicate you are in sexual prime
- Tops others with less make-up

- Tanned skin indicates an affluent lifestyle
- Waitresses get bigger tips if wearing make-up
- Want to impress
- You care what you look like
- You like the process of applying it

Reasons for not using make-up

- Approached less by strangers and guys without make-up which is good
- At menopause women lose water from skin due to their hot flushes.
- Can get used to my real face
- Can't be bothered sitting for hours in front of a mirror putting on make-up and taking it off again
- Can rely on personality for confidence i.e. how you act not what you look like
- Don't want to clog up the pores.
- Don't want to look like a clown

- If God wanted you to be different he would not have used make-up
- Postnatal skin changes
- Rebel against what is accepted and don't use it
- Rubbing eyes and sweating a lot means make-up can be spoilt
- Treated differently if you stop wearing make-up

4 SKIN DEEP

- The epidermis has five layers. Outside the stratified squamous is the stratum corneum. It is 10-20 micro metres thick and can be 25-30 layers of dead cells. The last layer of the epidermis is the stratum basale or germinatum.

- Outer stratum corneum is a barrier to many inorganic chemicals. There are three layers epidermis, dermis and hypodermis. The epidermis has no blood vessels. Cells move up after division and become filled with Kerstin they reach stratum corneum and are sloughed off.

- Skin is waterproof but there are ways for some chemicals to travel through the skin which includes between cells, through cells, through glands or hair bases or pores. The stratum corneum is like a brick wall with fat lipid cement. Many are dead cells with cement between the sheets. Protein joins cells together to form bridges. Solvents will dissolve cement enzymes and can affect what enters.

- Skin young and old is different. Skin around the eyes is thinner and sensitive and the first area to indicate ageing. Ageing produces thinner skin due to a loss of elasticity, less oil from glands and blood flow. Ageing skin includes sagging, wrinkles, redness, brown discoloration, yellowing and abnormal growths.

- There are three main skin types- oily, dry or a mixture of the two. You need to clean the skin thoroughly several times a week. Your glands are overactive. This results in oily, shiny, skin, which encourages spots and pimples although it is less prone to wrinkling. Oily skin stops moisture escaping but pores become blocked with dead cells which don't slough off easily pores are more visible

- Organic and inorganic chemicals can just remain on the surface, semi penetrate or penetrate the skin into the blood stream. They can also be used to remove dead skin or open up pores.

Examples of external treatments

- Jojoba oil is closest to our own sebum and is good for dry skin
- Honey enzymes can clear dead skin
- Fruit can be placed on faces and also cucumber which reduces inflammation
- Homemade recipes include curdled milk for acne
- There is a need to cleanse in the morning as well as night even if wearing no make-up. At night, the skin renews itself and cleansing and also removing make-up may prevent your skin becoming damaged this damaging you skin.
- Important not to overload make-up or your skin may look more puffy
- Can add fish scales to lipstick and eye shadow to make the eyes shimmer

- Prolonged leaving make-up on at night can lead to cysts, dry skin and flaky skin. It can also cause cracked lips and corners of the mouth, and enlarged pores and redness
- Sunblock uses titanium dioxide and is opaque
- Need to reapply sunscreen as it is still transparent.
- One can remove puffiness under the eyes by stroking down the side of the nose and the puffiness will move to the other side
- Vitamins A, D, C, and E help the skin. A helps keratisation. D is for the immune system while Vitamin C and E act as an antioxidants

Chemical penetration

- Skin can be permeable to lipids and fat solvents
- Some chemicals are absorbed into the bloodstream. Examples include sulphates, triclosans phthalates, stearic acid and benzene. Benzene can be carcinogenic

- There is better skin penetration by light with soluble chemicals than with ionic ones

- Lipid soluble substances can penetrate. Examples include hormones, vitamin D and K, phenol, nicotine, strychnine and sarin nerve gas. Diffusion can depend on many factors such as concentration, size of particles in a solution, temperature and area exposed.

- Pores push out hair and oil but as you age these pores can become larger

- To increase skin permeability-UV light damage of the skin surface weakens the boundary stratum corneum and epidermal layer and can allow nano particles in

- One can use tape to strip the thin top skin layer off or one can add chemicals to increase the permeability of oleic acid, and polyvinylpyrrolidone dimethyl sulfoxide

- Thai women were known to slap their cheeks to get rid of wrinkles

- Mercury is skin permeable. Molecule transfer depends on polarity, volatility, solubility, concentration, molecular weight, particle size and duration of the chemical on the skin

- Substances can penetrate e.g. oleic acid penetrates to the deep layers and allow oils and cleansers to enter.

- With time more nicotine can enter in low amounts. This can cause vomiting and illness.

- Water leaves epidermis layer through pores and can reverse direction also. i.e. in hydration. In the stratum corneum lipids are sandwiched between layers of dead cells so form a barrier.

- Nanoparticle spheres can diffuse or travel down follicles glands to reach the dermis layer Silver has no penetration but gold, zinc and titanium oxide can penetrate.

- Short high voltage electric pulses can increase permeability and charged molecules can enter. Patches can use nano medicine and drugs e.g. nicotine

- Polar molecules, e.g. menthol, attach to skin lipids and other end of the molecule to water so that menthol acts as a carrier.
- Foetal skin has better water and solute exchange between foetus and amniotic fluid during pregnancy.

<u>5 TECHNOLOGY STEPS IN</u>

- Electrically charged micro needles –can cause semi-permanent or permanent markings on the skin so that make-up or other products can enter the skin and modify or change the appearance of the skin.
- Electroporation- high charge short pulse so that micromolecules can enter
- Ionphoresis- uses charged electrodes which uses repulsion of equally charged carriers
- Microcircuit technology with a facial toner- targets the muscles. Daily use of an oil then a gel primer is added. One can first use different levels of intensity on toning the muscles of face. Targeting different areas of the face enhances condition through a micro current which tones strengthens and firms the muscles. It is possibly something worth trying before using a treatment with injections

- Microdermal abrasion- removes part of or an extensive amount of the upper surface of the skin to leave a smoother surface of younger cells. The abrasive can be aluminium oxide crystals or silica spheres moved by a rotating hand piece over the skin. This method gives better muscle tone, opens pores and can remove pigmentation with repeated treatments

- Nanotechnology- particles which are a billionth of a metre in diameter are used. Standards for use are still required .Nano emulsions of oil and water help to increase the content of nutritious oils which can contain vitamins or released from liposomes. They do not cross the skin barrier. Nano pigments can contain titanium dioxide and zinc oxide used in sunscreens so as to reflect sunlight. These do not cross the skin barrier and also exist in some toothpastes. Nanno carriers can liquidize the stratum corneum polysaccharide nanoparticles

- Photorejuvenation- a low energy treatment using light which produces heat to help remove wrinkles and lines. Increases blood flow and may improve tone.

- Phonophoresis sonophoresis uses ultrasound 20-100 KHz to produce small gas bubbles which collapse. As the skin is worn away chemicals pass in easier which increase lipid flow by the temperature increase.

- Stem cell science- stem cells from plants and animals are often used in ant-ageing products and are said to help regenerate the skin. However, cells in many products are no longer living, so using these does not have the effect used in other medical treatments. Plant cells can provide antioxidants but not the attributes that the plant would have in its normal growing environment. The use of extracts from plant stem cells, for example protein extracts has still to be fully established

- Micellar technology- is a form of skin cleanser which sticks to debris. It relies on a charged particle. One end loves water, the other hates it, but it likes soils and fats. On the face the tail end picks up the dirt and the oil on your face which can then be wiped off with cotton wool.

6 EXAMPLES OF TERMINOLOGY

- Abrasives-for dead skin removal. These can be gels lotions and creams. Abrasives include apricot kernel. beads, sea salt, sugar, groundnut shells, rice, bran and groundnut kernels.
- Acids –used for pH balance
- Agents for skin absorption- includes vitamin C, vitamin B, caffeine, hydroquinone and extracts from green teas or grape
- Ageing-from 30 years less collagen is present under the skin. The skin can lose firmness and wrinkles. Lines and sagging occur in the skin especially around the eyes
- Alcohol dilates blood vessels and can break them. It attacks fibres and dehydrates.
- Alcohol products are not recommended for sensitive skin
- Alkaline-helps neutralise pH. An example is sodium hydroxide,

- Anti-ageing cream- often a moisturiser commonly put on at night which prevents or covers up lines or wrinkles. Creams can protect against the aging effect of sunlight, help with cell growth, exfoliation, and increase antioxidants to prevent cell damage and relax muscles. They can contain collagen ,vitamin E and fruit acids in exfoliators

- Anti-inflammatory-prevents inflammation and reddening of skin, eg.acacia

- Anti-irritant – used for preventing skin irritation. Examples are green tea, and liquorice

- Antioxidants- these neutralise free radicals that kill skin cells. Also they help prevent colour loss and ensure ingredients remain active (some may be taken orally). Examples include vitamins C, A and E, lipoic acid, kinetin, apple fruit extract, barley extract, brazil nut extract and rose oil

- Antimicrobials-kill bacteria and fungi. Examples include aniseed, benzophenone chloride, and 1.2-hexanediol used on scabs
- Bee venom- the sting toxin increases blood flow to an area. This stimulates the production of collagen and elastin under the skin which drops at menopause causing wrinkles
- Binding agents- used to hold products together. Examples are wax, fat and gums
- Body butter-a thick substance with fatty oils also used as moisturiser. This is good for dry but not oily skins. An example is Shea butter.
- Botanicals- chemicals from natural plants which can regenerate the skin e.g. Aloe Vera.
- Botox- an extract from the botulism bacteria which produces neurotoxins causing muscle paralysis. It can potentially have other side effects including drooping eyebrows, etc.
- Blush- a powder, cream or gel which sculpts and slims the face. One can accentuate cheek

bones and forehead. It needs to be applied in one direction and it sculpts and slims the face

- Bronzer- can help make cheek bones stand out a little and can be used as a foundation.

- Chemical peels- chemicals that erode the upper layers of the skin to leave a smoother scar layer underneath depending on duration of application. This can affect the skin tone and sensitivity to ultraviolet light.

- Cleanser-facial cleansers, milk or cream help to moisturise, wipe off make-up etc. It can also be as a deep foaming lather and can include seaweed, tea tree or vitamin E

- Coenzyme Q10- is supposed to get rid of wrinkles by providing the cells with food.

- Colour corrector –to stop colours cancelling each other out.

- Concealers- cream for covering blemishes, imperfections, scars, spots, pimples or pigmentation hides imperfections scars pimples marks. Often the cream is thicker than foundation and lasts longer and can mould over skin. It can be used after foundation as can see imperfections but must be same shade as skin so that it will blend in

- Combination skin- has areas which are oily or dry. They need to be treated separately. Need to avoid rich moisturisers or oily ones
- Contouring-slims face, e.g. by using bronzing powder
- Creams- can help give depth to face and texture. Night cream is more hydrating and is heavier than day cream. Day cream-lighter texture and can be used under make-up and sunscreen
- Crow's feet-lines at the side of the eye, previously called 'laughter lines'. Now covered by make-up or Botox can be used
- Dermabrasion- removal of dead skin using silica or crystals for sensitive skin. Wire brushes can be used for deep peels but it is important to prevent exposure to infection or ultra violet light from sun.

- Dermal fillers- injections of silicon or collagen to remove lines or raise areas of the skin. Can cause allergic reactions.

- Dry skin-need to avoid using alcohol or soap, cream or milk cleansers. Remove dead skin and apply hydrating moisturisers

- Emollient – to soften or soothe the skin. Increases moisture barrier under the skin. Oils often fragrant, are used e.g. amyris, jojoba and sunflower. One can have non fragrant oils, e.g. avocado cocoa nut and cocoa butter

- Essential oil-oil from a plant, often fragrant and volatile

- Exfoliators –they remove dead skin and can be mildly acid or abrasive. Found in liquid or gel form. They can be derived from acetic acid, lactic, salicylic and glycolic acid

- Eye shadow -adds drama and depth to the eyes. Dark shadows around the eyes make the eyes appear to shrink or recede. Can be deepened using a wet brush.

- Exfoliant – for pH. balance e.g. ammonium chloride
- Eyelash curler-can be used to make the eyes look bigger. Can also put glitter under lower lashes.
- Eyelash comb-used on wet eyelashes to stop mascara clumping
- Eyeliner – liquid or soft pencil used to draw lines above and beneath the eye can elongate the size of the eye. White liner on eyes makes eyes look bigger and makes one look more awake. Drawing them pointing down can give a sad look but up at the sides gives a cat like look.
- Eye pencils – can be used on eyebrows to fill in the gaps. Can also be creams used to define eyelids
- Eye drops- can be used on bloodshot eyes to restrict vessels
- Face creams – huge range and functions, can be made from anything including meteorites

- Face masks - absorb oil and dust from skin. Can be clay or cotton masks soaked in serum and treatments. Can peel off and exfoliate skin

- Foundation is like a canvas, a base for other make-up. It can be cream, mousse, matte powder, liniment, creamy or oil. Can be used over a primer and can have various tones depending on skin type and needs and also as a concealer to cover blemishes and spots

- False eyelashes- can have different lengths and thicknesses. They need to match the natural lashes and can have a C or J curl. One may need to cut them to fit lid length before gluing on and then holding until set. Advised to leave 24 hours before applying mascara. Lashes can be waterproof and you can even swim wearing them

- Fillers -used to fill crevices in the skin to help smooth appearance. Common in anti-ageing creams

- Gels – can include glycerine and are often used at night on mature skin but can be used at any age. They can be softened with moisturisers. Brow gels keep eyebrows in shape.

- Hypoallergenics –chemicals usually not giving allergic reactions.

- Highlighter- a liquid cream or powder for emphasis of certain features, e.g. full cheeks

- Humectants attract water to skin from surroundings. e.g. Aloe Vera

- Hydrophilic dye promoters –e.g. pyrrolidones which go into hydrophobic regions and reduce the barrier function

- Increased penetration- sulphoxides dissolve salts and cause polar denaturation of structural protein. They also change alpha helix protein coil structure to the beta form

- Inorganic filter products have a range of sized particles that scatter and absorb UV

- Laser therapies- removes skin surface like dermal abrasion or dermal peels

- Lift and tighten-hydrates, tightens or firms skin and reduces dark circles under the eyes. Lighteners include mucopolysaccharides and hyaluronic acid

- Lip balm moisturisers can also have sunscreen included

- Lip gloss- gives clear or shiny appearance often with vaseline and can be scented or flavoured.

- Lip liner- for lip outlining make lips look bigger. They can be used outside natural lipline

- Lip smoothing-covers lines on lips by exfoliation and use of filler such as sugar beads for example.

- Liposomes- packets of fluid in cells which carry substances e.g. vitamins into cells

- Lipophilic substance- a transporter substance, e.g. propylene glycolterpenoids which work with penetration enhancers such as lipophilic drugs to increase fluidisation of hydrocarbon chains in skin

- Lip seal-seals in lipstick to help water proofing
- Lipsticks –emphasing lips, a temporary coat of lips water or gel based. Many colours and textures exist. Often natural shades are used in the day but brighter tones are used at night. They can be frosted or iridescent and excess can be removed by rolling finger around inside the lips
- Lotions-chemicals that moisturise and clean the skin
- Lubricants-chemicals that improve flow
- Make-up artist-a person involved in creativity and precision who understands the skin, its physiology and functions.
- Mascara-used on eyelashes for increasing the length. It can be any colour and waterproof. You need to apply anther coat before first is dry in order to increase the thickness of the eyelashes
- Mature skin cleanse- can use rich moisturisers and exfoliants. Use oil and water and anti-

ageing serums, antioxidants, vitamins and
sunscreen. Don't shift the skin too much
when cleansing

- Moisturiser -as creams lotions or gels. They
  can hydrate the skin so as to retain moisture.
  Can be applied before foundation. Can also
  be oil with herbs or chemicals included. Urea
  is a natural moisturiser which holds water.

- Micro lens pigments -ones which can diffuse
  light using various colours

- Micropigmentation-a permanent make-up that
  works by implanting hypoallergenic pigments
  into the skin surface. Used for eyebrow
  reconstruction, cleft lips white patches etc.

- Mineral make-up-is longer lasting and can be
  ant-inflammatory and good for sensitive skins.
  Examples include titanium oxide zinc and
  iron oxides. Minerals can also act as physical
  sunscreens and help prevent water loss.

- Natural face lift massage- uses exercises and
  pressure at standard sites on the face to help
  skin appear softer and brighter and toned

- Night cream-a moisturiser which helps regeneration of the skin during the night. Useful also to use as a moisturiser. It can contain substances to help collagen production and vitamins

- Nightingale poo facial. –this uses Japanese bush warbler faeces as an exfoliator. Contains amino acid guanine a bleaching agent and urea as a humectant. It lightens dark areas of the face and tightens skin

- Oily skin-should use non oily products, lavender oil for spots, foaming cleansers and clay mask to absorb oil.

- Oestrogen- the female hormone in women which gives a prominent bone structure compared to men. Women may want to change this with make-up

- Organic filter products- these absorb ultraviolet light and change it to heat

- Penetrants-can enter the skin, examples include caffeine which reduce redness Penetration enhancers –help penetration. A lipophilic enhancer can be produced by adding propylene glycol and ethanol. This disturbs lipid packing order in skin. An example is ethyl acetate

- Placental face mask topping- dried human placenta used in China for centuries. Said to boost collagen production and tightens skin for anti-ageing

- Plasticisers -stop the product cracking on the skin and give some stretch

- Plucking eye brows-This can take six weeks to recover or hairs may not grow back at all. It can be painful and time consuming and over plucking can alter your looks. Moving hair between the eyes make them look further apart and your nose bigger

- Phyto minerals bioactive-these can contain many minerals and trace element contained in plant extracts and algae, often deposited millions of years ago.

- Polisher action cleaner-removes dead skin cells and scars and wrinkles. It also nourishes the skin so that skin looks lighter and glows.

- Porosity- is the amount of entry through skin. This can be increased using the alcohol ethanol. Also found in patches where the chemical extracts the lipids and proteins

- Preservatives-prevent or slow down microbial of fungal growth in products and may also stabilise the products anti-oxidants. Examples include tea tree oil and potassium sorbate

- Primers -reduce pore size and are used before eye shadow or foundation. Primers help make-up cling to skin better and longer

- Protective layer- placed on top of make-up

- Puffiness and dark eye circles-often caused with ageing. Examples of a chemical used to reduce this is caffeine which restricts blood flow

- Retinols-from vitamin A, an antioxidant which protects in sun

- Rouge -as powder, liquid or cream used to bring out colour and promote cheek bones

- Self-tanning- as moisturiser or an all-round spray tan applied in a cubicle.

- Sensitive skin-one that reacts to chemicals. You may need to cut down on the use of chemicals and reduce alcohol. Check cleaners, toners for contents. Avoid colours and preservatives and choose hypoallergenic products. Check ingredients on packets

- Separate phases in bilayer lipids –unsaturated fatty acids, examples include oleic, lauric, linoleic and caprylic acids

- Serum –hydrates and often used before moisturiser. Can contain pure ingredients. Dry and stiff skin needs moisturiser on top. Often used at night where serum is more concentrated.

- Skin types-oily, dry or a combination of these over different areas of face. Also sensitive and maturing skin

- Smoking -nicotine constricts the blood vessels, giving skin a greyish colour. Acetaldehyde will attack the skin fibres. Can make you look ten years older

- Solvents- a liquid used to dissolve chemicals. Water is the universal solvent but some chemicals are not water soluble so need other liquids to dissolve them. Examples include acetone or alcohols

- Spot sticks-used to apply antiseptic for blemishes etc. May contain witch hazel or tea tree oil

- Spreaders -can reduce surface tension and help with wetting and penetration of skin giving good surface cover.

- Subscision therapy—a probe placed into skin layers under a scar or wrinkle to initiate self-healing or production of more collagen to remove the defect

- Surfactants -foaming detergents to remove oils. Often non-ionic used which are good if they are similar to bilayer lipids

- Super food –may contain enzymes for preparation
- Tallow – chemical in make-up from animal fat carcasses
- Tanning- causes browning of skin. Tanning agents can be temporary creams or sprays which attach to proteins Face tans are lighter than body tans and dry skin takes in a higher concentration so it tans darker.
- Tan accelerator-helps increase melanin production in skin

- Thickening agents – to increase viscosity of products. Include aluminium oxide, arrow root, alkyl benzoate and ethyl hexyl palminate.
- Toners- help clog up your pores so some other make-up won't embed. Examples include witch-hazel salicylic acid and benzoyl peroxide for oily skins. In order to get the right skin pH for dry skin one needs to use alcohol free toners
- Translucent-see through application

- Vampire facial-uses your own blood plasma with platelets. Can also add fillers. Been used successfully for injuries and after burns. Now also used for anti-ageing. Plasma is Injected into skin

- Vitamin C -helps reduce sun damage and inflammation. It acts as an antioxidant and anti-ageing chemical.

- Waxing-to remove hair, after eye brow removal etc. After waxing one needs to take care of anti-ageing creams or other chemicals effects on the skin

- Water solubility-dissolves in water to different extents. A good example is urea but this is not very stable

- Weather- cold weather destroys the fat that stops the skin drying out

- Wrinkles-exposure to the sun can cause them. During hot weather more oil is produced from glands in the skin

7 ROLES NEEDING MAKE-UP

- The Wadaabe tribe from the Sahel desert, Niger chad were nomadic cattle herders. At the wife stealing festival (a salt festival). They make up their faces with black exaggerated lips and eyebrows. They put a white stripe down their nose with white spots on face and blacken their eyelids. They are polygamous and take each other's women but have to attract them with their make-up, face expressions such as rolling their eyes. They also show their teeth and dance wearing various adornments such as beaded hair and feathers. Men in this tribe have mirrors. Women can have facial scars and tattoos. Their make-up is from colourful desert plants

- George Washington sometimes wore make-up, even lipstick on some occasions

- In the 18th century more men than women in some places were using make-up.

- Indian face paint as well as holding magical powers was used to make Indians more ferocious. Different colours can be as lines or symbols on faces. Red can indicate a war paint while white peace. However yellow can indicate death or a hero. The designs painted were believed to hold magic powers for protection. Colours and images were also used to make the warriors, chiefs and braves look more ferocious. There were so many tribes of Native American Indians it is only possible to generalise the most common meanings of the colours and patterns of war paint, body paint or face paint.

- Military camouflage in tribes was used to strike fear into enemy. North American tribes, African and South America peoples commonly used such paint on their faces

- Tribal make up was seen as a badge for status in community. Tattooing on faces was common in Maori and Thai people. Small branding or skin injury is common in some African tribes

- On stage make-up includes on males in a theatrical role. White-faced actors exist in Japanese theatre. Geisha girls have white foundation with charcoal eyes and red lips shaped like that of a flower when fully trained. They also it is said use nightingale faeces to diminishes wrinkles and as a good defoliator

- Prostitutes wore excessive make-up to try to make them look younger

- Appearance in public calls for the use of make-up. Such people include celebrities, princesses, famous actresses and singers. Anyone on television or films is expected to be made-up to make them look more attractive.

- Children's face paints provide a huge range of forms including animals

- Clowns have different kinds of standard make-up. One kind is the white faced Joseph Grimaldi with eyebrows black, facial features black and red based on Pierrot. These are called harlequinade clowns. Another kind was used by Tom Belling Senior, the red clown or Auguste character. The nose is red with white around the eyes. The base features are increased with red and black and the mouth painted white. The third kind is Hobo tramp clown who has a pink or tan face and can have white around the eyes and mouth

- Morticians have to cover a large range of skin conditions and damage. The skin is cold and damp with death so they need highly pigmented creams which sets in powder and is absorbed into the upper layers of the skin. Silica gel can be used for damaged skin and then camouflage make-up is placed over this. For lips and eyebrows they have cosmetic staining pens to ensure colour is not lost and lipstick can be applied after. Normal make-up can be put over the camouflage base.

8 CLAIMS TO PROMOTE MAKE-UP USE

Often claims are not true, trust is abused and bits of information are left out

- A bronzer eye shadow palette
- A clinical product so no need for a fancy smell
- A recognised lifting product
- Accepted by the skin
- Activity like a magnet draws out make-up
- Advertised in an up market magazine
- Allow yourself a little luxury
- Anti-ageing as titanium dioxide included
- Anti-ageing ingredients
- Award winning
- Based on science so you can trust it
- Becoming more precious with time
- Been around for 10-20 years so must be good
- Boost skin fragrance

- Boost to transforming the skin
- Can mix highlighter with foundation
- Catch that moment
- Change your life
- Chemical free (but water is a chemical)
- Chromatogram measures efficiency of the oils and does not look fake
- Clearer skin
- Completely portable
- Contains many antioxidants
- Does not stain clothes or bed linen at night
- Easy to use on a plane
- Faces looking radiant
- Fantastic hydration
- Feels like it is doing something
- Feels like luxury
- Firming and toning by using vitamin E
- Formulations of this product are for different skin types
- Fresh natural bronzing natural radiance
- Fresh raspberry seed oil for nourishing

- Full nourishing gel
- Give a healthy glow
- Give it a whirl
- Give unique texture
- Give you confidence
- Gives a fresh finish
- Gives skin a raidiancy
- Good surface dehydration
- Gradual glow
- Great brands
- Has a popcorn effect on line and wrinkles holds onto moisture
- Has ironing effect on wrinkles
- Has lifelong beauty
- Has neuropeptides with carrier
- Hassle free
- High potency
- Highlighted look
- Humectants stop the product drying out
- Ideal for gifting to have as a present for someone

- Improves quality of skin
- Instant results five minute entry
- Laboratory built especially to make ingredients
- Last longer e.g., cochineal
- Lasts for two years keeps on going
- Light as a feather
- Limited stock
- Lip smoothing
- Long money back guarantee
- Look more refreshed with mascara and lipstick
- Displayed with a clinical style presentation on shelves for different skin types
- Make you appear better
- Many million bottles sold in other countries
- Masters art and science
- Melts into the skin
- Men look longer at someone with make-up on especially if they have red lipstick
- Mimics the sunshine

- More natural so the more preservatives are included
- Most firming for skin
- Neutral
- Nine till four spray
- Not so creamy so won't clog up pores
- Now flowers are not allowed in hospital. Fragrances are important. Make-up with scent is therefore important
- Numbers in the top ten
- Oils the skin
- Organic
- pH. balanced
- Powerful science
- Primer binds moisture into the lashes also good for lengthening and thickening mascara
- Produces baby like skin (placental face mask)
- Pseudoscientific claims about not being tested on animals
- Removes any make-up
- Renew your skin

- Results look natural
- Retextures your skin
- Safer tan avoids burn
- Saves money
- Scent in make-up is so important
- Sceptical claims can include products are natural, organic, fragrance free, preservative free and hypoallergenic
- Silky so rich and light
- Skin dynamically revitalised
- Skin like a trampoline
- Smells delicious and smell is tied to memory association.
- Smoothing e.g. for mascara. Coconut oil won't stay smooth
- Softer skin
- Strong enough to cover a tattoo
- Sucks out impurities solubises them
- Tans contrast white make-up
- This is a real treatment
- Tingling means it's working

- To use when the skin hot and lush so needs refreshing
- Totally unique
- Travel bag perfect
- Travel size plump firm
- Use for bruises
- Uses advice from an ophthalmologist
- UV light activates enzymes and repairs DNA and preserves collagen structure
- Voted for by industry experts
- Waterproofs top coat weather proofs
- Why should you be the odd one out
- Won't come off when swimming
- Working with a University in a major country. Covers and prevents pigmentation
- Working with celebrities on the product development
- Working with expert gardeners to develop botanicals

9 DANGERS OF MAKE-UP AND LEGISLATION

- Minerals in make-up today are purer and less toxic than in the past.

- Some ingredients in make-up can cause irritation, allergies, cancers and can affect internal organs.

- Cosmetics should not affect skin metabolism i.e. collagen production Never leave on too long and wash off at night

- Can't read the entire label when you buy it. It may contain over twenty ingredients

- Synthetic preservatives such as parabens and some dyes can trigger cancers

- Titanium dioxide use in foundation and other products is believed to show no evidence of having harmful effects but the particles may be coated with other chemicals in some preparations

- Belladonna was used by the Romans is used to dilate pupils. It is poisonous

- Talc was used as a filler in the past and may have had traces of asbestos
- Aluminium in lipsticks can cause anaemia, respiratory disease if consumed. Some lipstick colours cause allergic reactions so non allergenic colours were developed, e.g. silver
- Twentieth century thiomersla is made from mercury and causes poisoning
- Aloe Vera was not accepted in make-up previously but has always been used to calm sensitive skin
- Every time you apply make-up eventually the skin absorbs it and this can cause irritation and premature ageing
- Expensive anti-ageing creams can have little or no effect
- Anti-ageing products can be made from placental facial stem cells from a sheep's placenta. It can increase collagen. Also sperm and cryotherapy have been tried

- Bacteria breed in eyeliners and mascara. Make-up brushes often have dirt and bacteria clinging to them

- Preservatives prevent bacteria and yeasts and there are strict rules on their use. If no preservatives were present these products would spoil. Products from natural sources give an open jar symbol fruit and plant extracts have preservatives

- Oil based make-up can cause acne, blackheads and blocks pores especially if the skin is oily.

- Applying eyeliner to inside lash line can affect the eyes. Mascara can block oil producing pores along the length and lash line of eyelid and one can get red eyes

- The kind and amount of make-up used can link you to a social category It can even signal aggressiveness or sexuality but less so now

- Still a feeling exists that make-up is frowned upon by members of the church and some part of society, so the aim to make it look more natural and less threatening

- One can fall into a make-up palette and end up looking like clown while using too many chemicals
- Over half the cosmetics have the female hormone oestrogen in them that can disrupt hormones in the body
- Foundation as a liquid, can only last six months as does mascara before being out of date
- Leaving mascara on at night can cause eye lashes to dry and fall out, and using a curler with mascara also can break hairs
- Some cosmetic companies can have little if any regulations
- US food and drug administration regulations mainly apply to the body. Make-up is for cleansing, beautifying and promoting attractiveness without affecting the body's structure or functions. Soap is not included in this.

- EU regulations list substances listed not to be used in make-up. Clarification is mainly based on the pure form of the chemical

- Different countries in the European Union have different definitions of organic and natural but all cosmetics are chemicals as is water

- Chemical safety is often directed at colourings, preservatives and ultraviolet filtering properties

- Controversial ingredients include those derived from petrol, sodium lauryl sulphate (a surfactant), parabens and phalates which may cause dermatitis. At low levels they may be deemed safe

The following is an example of a typical cleansing mousse on sale today for sensitive skin which has 21 constituents Ingredients:

1 solvent-water

3 Humectants- take in water

2 Surfactant cleansers

1 Thickener and foam booster from coconut oil

1 Penetrant

1 Acid to adjust acid base level

3 Preservatives antimicrobials

1Lubricant and for hydration

2 Emulsifiers and emollient

1 Binding agent

3 Antioxidants anti-ageing

1 Keratin synthesis activator

1 Alkali to control pH

<u>10 FAMOUS SAYINGS</u>

- Audrey Hepburn-"Make-up can only make you look pretty on the outside, but it doesn't help if you're ugly on the inside, unless you eat the make-up"
- Calvin Klein –"The best thing is to look natural but it takes make-up to look natural"
- Coco Chanel-"The best colour in the whole world is the one that looks good on you!"
- Courtney summers –"My dad used the world to say make-up was a shallow girls sport but it's not"
- Dolly Parton-" It costs a lot of money to money to look this cheap"
- Elizabeth Taylor –"Pour your drink, put on some lipstick and pull yourself together"
- Lady Gaga –"Whether I'm wearing lots of make-up or no make-up I'm the same person inside"

- Marilyn Monroe- "Beneath the make-up and behind the smile I am just a girl who wishes for the world"
- Miss Piggy -(Muppets)-"Beauty is in the eye of the beholder and it may be necessary from time to time to give a stupid or misinformed beholder a black eye"
- Sophia Lauren- "Beauty is how you feel inside and it reflects in your eyes. It is not something physical"
- Sophia Loren –"Nothing makes a woman more beautiful than the belief that she is beautiful"
- Yves Saint Laurent-"The most beautiful make-up of a woman is passion. But cosmetics are easier to buy"

Make-up in films

Academy awards exist for best make-up by academy of motion pictures and sciences. Example include-

- Bram Stokers Dracula

- The Fly
- Wizard of Oz (The original tin man was allergic to make-up and was replaced)
- Edward Scissor Hands, Johnny Depp. Stan Winston found that a white face enhanced the scars on the face of Edward
- The Incredible Melting Man. Rick baker used syrup and paint for the melting effect
- Planet of the Apes. John Chambers was an expert prosphetic make-up artist who created the apes

11 FIVE MAIN POINTS ABOUT MAKE-UP

You don't need make-up to be beautiful. Beauty still remains in the eye of the beholder. You need to believe you're beautiful. You may look awful with no make-up but with minimal make-up you may still look different to employers and friends but you will have a more natural look

2. Most people look at inner beauty not physical attractiveness when they choose their partner. It is said in Genesis in the Christian Bible that we all were created in the image of God, so looking at someone else you could be looking at God who is perfect in every way.

3. Beauty is skin deep. Healthy skin is what you really need to look beautiful. A cleanser, facial scrub and moisturiser can rejuvenate your face. You don't need lipstick if your lips are well looked after and you can still use a pale gloss or vaseline. To help keep your skin healthier antioxidants in food in your diet in reasonable proportions will help with this, plus drinking plenty of water every day

4. Beware of the claims made by manufacturers and salespeople in the media and in magazines. Complicated chemical names and novel contents such as exotic fruits and metals such as gold are all there to impress. Read the packaging before buying, the more chemicals in the product then the less natural he product is.

5. Test out products first to ensure that they don't cause allergies initially, or have the potential to do so after repeated use. Ask others about your appearance. Styles change so find the make-up you are happy to live with and which gives you confidence, makes you feel ready to face the world outside and is not just something you routinely slap on your face every day as a habit.

Other booklets in the really, really, really useful series include:

1. How to be a Successful Business Weed
2. How to Deal with Life's Snakes and Ladders
3. Pens for Pops
4. How to be a successful charity shop
6. Know Your Students and Build Your Image

Other books by Mike Pearce:

1. Pattern for Purpose- God's and Man's designs
2. Red Fred Cell and Friends
3. Human Termites eat London
4. Pigeons Splat London
5. Glass Anemones Tentacle-ize London
6. Tuppeny Hangover
7. I am Termite
8. The littlest Oyster
9. Bits and Bobs
10. The Shell Man
11. Cats at Christmas
12. Tails, Tales
13. Trust-Nothing but a Must
14. In a Dark, Dark Corner was the Holy Ghost
15. The shell lady
16. Captain Grottbuster versus the Grey World
17. London's Nemesis(Trilogy of 3,4 and 5 above
18. Saved by Angels (Trilogy of 6,8 and 14 above)
19. The World of Wax

ABOUT THE AUTHOR

Dr Mike Pearce is a scientist interested in behaviour. He also was a lecturer in human biology and health at a college in Canterbury, Kent.